1001 Things It Means to Be a Dad

(Some Assembly Required)

HARRY H. HARRISON JR.

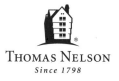

THOMAS NELSON
Since 1798

NASHVILLE   DALLAS   MEXICO CITY   RIO DE JANEIRO   BEIJING

Table of Contents

Introduction

Men handle the whole baby thing differently than women do.

Upon hearing the news, they don't go to the office, burst into tears, and scream, "We're pregnant!" They don't stay up late at night reading books on lactation. They think buying a baby crib just about wraps up the whole shopping thing. They are flabbergasted to learn that a baby has needs. And they think that by going to birthing class and learning the word *push*, they've become active participants, if not authority figures, in the pregnancy world.

But, of course, a man can't help but notice the two thousand books stacked up on his wife's bedside table or discover that he can actually feel a baby's foot inside her stomach, or that whenever she wants to talk about the baby, there's usually one minute left in the game and his team is driving for the go-ahead touchdown, so he has to act interested while secretly wishing she would move just two inches to the left so he can see the TV.

The fact is, dads are just as excited, depressed, worried, happy, awed, and stressed as moms, but who do they tell this to? Their workout buddies? Fat chance. Yet, that's exactly who they should be talking to. Other men. Other dads. Other dads-to-be. So this book is like telling a bunch of other guys, "Uh . . . we're . . . uh . . . having a baby and . . . and I'm feeling, you know, kind of weird."

And his friends look at him sympathetically, and one of them says, "Really? Because that's the way you're gonna feel for the rest of your life. But at least your kids will think you know what you're doing. For a while." •

Dad Rules

1. Being a dad means
becoming heroic.

•

2. Being a dad means being
a man. In all situations.

•

3. Being a dad means understanding
God has big plans for you. He chose
you to be the father of His child.

•

4. Being a dad means making
promises—and keeping them.

5. Being a dad means being around. Studies show that kids without responsible fathers are more likely to experience poverty, perform poorly in school, and engage in criminal activity, premarital sex, drug abuse, and heavy alcohol consumption.

•

6. Being a dad means admitting your screw-ups, but not dwelling on them.

•

7. Being a dad means providing for your family. And that can mean sleepless nights, ulcers, and low-grade fear.

8. Being a dad means
making your child feel safe.

•

9. Being a dad means
telling them a little blood
won't hurt them.

•

10. Being a dad means
telling your kids to deal
with scrapes and bruises by:

A. "Walk it off!"
B. "Blow on it."
C. "Run it under cold water."

11. Being a dad means telling stories
of adventure and bravery.

12. Being a dad means
assuring Mom that growing up
involves pain and suffering.

13. Being a dad means teaching
that happiness isn't a goal,
but a consequence.

14. Being a dad means having
high expectations for your kids.

15. Being a dad means being the heavy. It's your job to say no.

•

16. Being a dad means being your child's father. Not your child's friend. Dads who get this confused have confused kids.

•

17. Being a dad means demanding peace over justice. No matter who hit whom last.

•

18. Being a dad means teaching your kids that life is unfair.

19. Being a dad means making your kids believe they can do it themselves.

•

20. Being a dad means realizing if you don't want to move into a six-bedroom house, you need a vasectomy.

•

21. Being a dad means showing them how to stand up for their rights.

•

22. Being a dad means understanding that food stolen off your plate tastes better to your kids than any other food in the world.

23. Being a dad means showing your kids how to fix stuff. It helps, of course, if you know how to fix stuff.

•

24. Being a dad means you have to get off the couch.

•

25. Being a dad means giving your kids courage.

•

26. Being a dad takes balls— baseballs, footballs, soccer balls, dodge balls, basketballs, tennis balls, and other spherical or semispherical objects.

27. Being a dad means teaching your kids to stand on their own two feet. Literally and philosophically.

28. Being a dad means letting them live without being the center of attention all the time.

29. Being a dad means making sure you live in a neighborhood safe enough for kids.

30. Being a dad means having more confidence in your kids than they have in themselves.

31. Being a dad means realizing that the only way to avoid sibling rivalry is to avoid siblings.

32. Being a dad means realizing life doesn't get any better than this. Ever.

33. Being a dad means understanding how dumb you are depends on the age of your child:

0 to 6 years old
Dad knows everything.

6 to 8 years old
Dad knows almost everything.

8 to 12 years old
Dad knows many things.

12 to 16 years old
Dad knows one or two things.

16 to 20 years old
Dad knows nothing.

20 to 23 years old
Maybe Dad does know
one or two things.

23 to 25 years old
Actually, Dad knows many things.

Over 25
Dad knows everything.

Fathers-to-Be

34. Being a dad means secretly panicking after hearing the news your wife's pregnant, accompanied by feelings of nausea, doom, and the need to hold on to the remote control.

•

35. Being a dad means showing unrestrained joy at the color of her urine.

•

36. Being a dad means realizing one of the most important things you can do for your baby is to love his mother.

37. Being a dad means
determining to influence your
child's faith, morals, integrity, and
convictions before society does.

•

38. Being a dad means praying for
your wife and child—ceaselessly.

•

39. Being a dad means
being a good husband.
Kids never have a good divorce.

•

40. Being a dad means learning
it takes some $285,000 to raise a
child and thinking you're screwed.

41. Being a dad means believing
you have about two weeks to get
all this figured out—and then,
eighteen years later, realizing you
still don't have it all figured out.

•

42. Being a dad means listening
to your father and your father-in-law
talk about raising kids, regardless
of what kind of fathers they were.

•

43. Being a dad means realizing
you'll see your wife's body again
in about fifteen months.

44. Being a dad means
discovering that living with
a pregnant woman is a lot like
living with a woman with PMS.
Only she's heavier, moodier, and the
symptoms don't go away in a week.

•

45. Being a dad means buying
your unborn baby a baseball
glove while everyone else is buying
teething toys and baby mobiles.

•

46. Being a dad means waking up
in a cold sweat over the thought of
your increased responsibility. This is
called "delayed onset maturity."

47. Being a dad means
striking up conversations about
strollers with men at the gym.

•

48. Being a dad means figuring
out how a household can go from
being a two-person family supported
by two people to being a three-
person family supported by one.

•

49. Being a dad means giving
up motorcycling and parachuting.
You now have responsibilities.

•

50. Being a dad means
painting your media room pink
because it's now the nursery.

51. Being a dad means asking your wife's doctor how many babies he has delivered and wondering if that's enough experience.

•

52. Being a dad means never missing an appointment with the ob-gyn, especially in the beginning.

•

53. Being a dad means touring the maternity ward with your wife— all the while keeping a vigilant eye out for the vending machines.

54. Being a dad means finding out what the health insurance will pay. Some babies cost a big-screen TV. Some cost a small car.

•

55. Being a dad means thinking baby furniture means small prices because, really, how expensive could that small stuff be?

•

56. Being a dad means paying attention to life insurance commercials. And actually buying some.

57. Being a dad means sitting up alone at night looking at the MasterCard bill and realizing that, in every sense of the word, you're just getting started.

•

58. Being a dad means deciding only the best crib will do for your baby—and then, after pricing out cribs, wondering just how important a crib really is.

•

59. Being a dad means believing you can put a crib together, opening the box to find two thousand parts and eight pages of instructions, and then, after six hours, realizing you're missing the three most critical pieces.

60. Being a dad means finally getting the crib together at 6:00 a.m. only to learn you need to spend more money. On a mattress. Actually, on two of them.

•

61. Being a dad means telling your wife how blessed your child is to have her for a mother.

•

62. Being a dad means asking God to make you the kind of father He wants you to be.

•

63. Being a dad means celebrating the fact she's beginning to show.

64. Being a dad means giving your wife the side of the bed near the bathroom. She'll be peeing most of the night.

•

65. Being a dad means dealing with a 2:30 a.m. food craving for cottage cheese with french dressing and chili peppers. And trying not to gag while your wife gulps it down next to you in bed.

•

66. Being a dad means waking up late at night just to play with your still-in-the-womb baby. Then once you get it rocking and rolling and kicking, you kiss your wife, roll over, and go to sleep.

67. Being a dad means realizing that last month's maternity clothes don't necessarily fit this month's maternity body.

•

68. Being a dad means finding out your once dainty flower of femininity now passes gas like a linebacker. The dog can get up and leave, but you can't.

•

69. Being a dad means talking to other men in restrooms about baby names.

•

70. Being a dad means thinking, *How hard could it be to name a baby?*

71. Being a dad means learning that arguing with a pregnant woman is suicidal.

•

72. Being a dad means quietly airing out the house after your wife takes her prenatal vitamins.

•

73. Being a dad means watching her breasts become those of a movie star. Of course you can't touch them.

•

74. Being a dad means not wanting to kill a good Saturday afternoon attending a baby shower—and then being consumed by guilt after your wife breaks down in tears crying, "This is your baby too!"

75. Being a dad means rubbing her back every night until the baby is born or your hands fall off, whichever comes first.

•

76. Being a dad means telling her she looks better with thin hair.

•

77. Being a dad means asking a clerk at every baby store to turn the TV to ESPN.

•

78. Being a dad means rubbing her belly with cocoa butter at night. (Depending on how nauseous she is, this may or may not lead anywhere.)

79. Being a dad means watching other men with their kids. And deciding which dads you want to imitate.

80. Being a dad means flying home on the red-eye so you can be at the ultrasound scan the next morning.

81. Being a dad means paying down all the debt you've piled up till now. It's easy enough to do since your wife doesn't feel like eating or leaving the house.

82. Being a dad means feeling overcome at the third month when you learn your baby is four inches long and weighs one ounce; has arms, hands, fingers, feet, and toes; and can open and close her fists and mouth and suck her thumb. The circulatory and urinary systems are even working. She's alive!

83. Being a dad means reading the sports section to your wife's stomach.

84. Being a dad means
reassuring a panic-stricken
mom at 3:00 a.m. that you have
a plan for the family finances
and to go back to sleep. (It helps
greatly here to actually have a plan.)

85. Being a dad means TiVoing
through any TV commercial with
a baby knowing that failure to do
so will result in ten minutes of tears.

86. Being a dad means telling your wife
she's going to be a great mom. Often.

87. Being a dad means coming home from work early just so you can push on her stomach and have your baby push back.

•

88. Being a dad means discovering that all moms have a deep genetic need to whack off all their hair. When this happens, tell her she looks great.

•

89. Being a dad means saying, "Good morning" and "Good night" to your wife's stomach. Perfectly normal.

90. Being a dad means trying to decide whether to calmly fill out the myriad of hospital and insurance forms now instead of watching *24*, or to wait and do so furiously right after your wife's water breaks all over the admissions room floor. It's not an easy call.

·

91. Being a dad means finding yourself nauseous, gaining weight, and feeling a bit moody. You have sympathetic pregnancy. Resist the urge to cut off all your hair.

92. Being a dad means learning your cologne that used to lead your wife to frisky behavior now causes her to barf.

•

93. Being a dad means standing in the grocery store aisle reading the nutritional label on baby food jars.

•

94. Being a dad means finding your wife—a fierce trial lawyer during the day—staying up all night cross-stitching a quilt for the nursery. This is called "nesting." Don't interfere.

95. Being a dad means discovering underwear twice the size of yours in the washing machine and not making a single comment.

•

96. Being a dad means getting the child-care question settled before the third month of pregnancy. Is your wife staying home? Can one of the grandmothers help with child care? What's the best child-care facility in your area?

97. Being a dad means visiting child-care providers. Asking questions. Calling references. This is one of the single most important issues you need resolved.

•

98. Being a dad means spending the last couple months of pregnancy watching videos of complete strangers giving birth. (This would probably be an excellent time to fill out those hospital forms.)

99. Being a dad means calling about nursery and private-school admission requirements. It's insane, but parents are enrolling their soon-to-be-born kids now.

•

100. Being a dad means being screamed at because your wife hates being pregnant. Agree with her.

•

101. Being a dad means worrying if her body will ever return to normal. It will. Maybe not totally, but 99.9 percent. Okay, 97 percent. Whatever.

102. Being a dad means making a budget and listing diapers, baby food, clothes, high chair, doctor's visits, etc., before you get to the poker night fund.

•

103. Being a dad means having scintillating dinner discussion about her hemorrhoid problems.

•

104. Being a dad means telling her she's beautiful even if she is the size of a barn. She needs to hear it.

105. Being a dad means worrying about the health of your wife and your unborn child.

•

106. Being a dad means wondering if this cell phone call means "Come get me!"

•

107. Being a dad means hearing scratching noises coming from the other side of the bed at night—and learning that itching becomes even more of a problem later in pregnancy.

108. Being a dad means taking your wife out as often as she feels like going out. Going out will soon be a memory.

•

109. Being a dad means appreciating her fragile condition when she says she doesn't think ten blankets, seven sheets, two cribs, one layette, seven mobiles, two changing tables, baby furniture, push toys, pull toys, and two chests of clothes will be enough. Go baby shopping with her again.

110. Being a dad means trying not to freak out when your baby's due date comes and goes and there's no baby. Only 5 percent actually arrive on time.

111. Being a dad means pricing out a Volvo or an SUV because side-impact safety protection suddenly matters to you.

112. Being a dad means trying to decide between a Bugaboo and a 42" plasma TV. Your wife, of course, has already decided.

113. Being a dad means not commenting when it feels like a whale just got into bed with you.

•

114. Being a dad means planning what to do when your wife goes into labor. What will happen if you're out of town? or she's in a meeting? Don't wait till contractions are coming every three minutes to make these decisions.

115. Being a dad means making plans in case of a C-section. It happens 20 percent of the time. (Will you, for instance, go with your wife to recovery or spend an hour alone with your baby? You need a plan.)

116. Being a dad means making sure you don't have to stop for gas during a midnight run to the hospital.

117. Being a dad means panicking at the first sign of labor only to learn it's false, feeling a bit worried at the second sign of labor only to learn it, too, is false, and then being on the golf course when your wife calls because she's in labor for the third time and wondering if you should answer the phone.

•

118. Being a dad means accepting the fact that your wife will probably go into labor late at night at least three times. This is just a preview of what children do to their parents' sleep.

119. Being a dad means wondering
if you should panic over the
labor contractions now or if
you can just wait until the end of
24 and then race to the hospital.

120. Being a dad means
asking your wife if she'd like to listen
to rock music or a sports station
on the way to the hospital.

121. Being a dad means trying to
time contractions while driving to
the hospital with her screaming,
"Drive faster!" in your ear.

122. Being a dad means realizing
your usefulness in the labor
room rivals that of a lampshade.
But you can be supportive.

123. Being a dad means learning
your baby is coming in an hour and
deciding maybe you ought to thumb
through a few of those child-care
books. Maybe fill out some forms.

124. Being a dad means staying calm
while you're in the delivery room.
If you have to throw up, go outside.

125. Being a dad means giving up the fantasy that you will be able to fix your wife's labor pains. Only the delivery of the baby can do that.

126. Being a dad means sitting in the labor room in the dark and listening to Pavarotti.

127. Being a dad means sneaking a peek at your Blackberry to see if you have any important e-mails. And, okay, to check the sports updates.

128. Being a dad means asking questions of the doctors and nurses all the time. Questions like "Do you know what you're doing?"

•

129. Being a dad means feeling guilty because you forgot the aroma oils that she says are the only things that will help reduce her pain.

•

130. Being a dad means listening to a woman—who has vowed for nine months that she wants natural childbirth—scream for pain relief after ten minutes of hard labor. It's okay. Her doctors won't be surprised.

131. Being a dad means confusing your wife's childbirth pain with her being in medical distress. She's miserable. But it's not Code Blue.

•

132. Being a dad means holding your wife's hand for five hours because she asks you to. Even if your hand turns white and loses all feeling.

•

133. Being a dad means reassuring her often that all is well.

•

134. Being a dad means gently telling your wife to push while she's shrieking for you to shut the hell up. True bonding.

135. Being a dad means being
asked to cut the umbilical cord.

•

136. Being a dad means sneaking
a camera phone into the delivery
room without your wife knowing it.

•

137. Being a dad means taking
a picture that causes her to
scream every time she sees it.

•

138. Being a dad means not being
able to put your newborn baby down.

Baby Dads

139. Being a dad means counting fingers and toes after delivery. Somebody has to.

•

140. Being a dad means posting five hundred photos of the birth, the mother, the baby, and the happy family on Flickr.

•

141. Being a dad means filling your wife's room with flowers. Not filling a vase. Filling her room.

•

142. Being a dad means realizing that more than a baby has been born. So has a father.

143. Being a dad means taking your newborn into the hospital chapel and offering your baby to God.

•

144. Being a dad means phoning brothers, sisters, distant aunts—everyone—the day the baby arrives. If anyone is left out, feelings will be hurt.

•

145. Being a dad means finding out how long the insurance company will allow your wife to stay in the hospital. And insisting she stay there and rest until the last possible minute.

146. Being a dad means asking
a nurse to show you how to change
your baby's diaper. This lesson will
give you the illusion of knowledge.

•

147. Being a dad means applying
for a Social Security number when
filling out your baby's birth certificate.
It's quick and easy—and you'll
need it to claim her as a deduction.

•

148. Being a dad means handling
with care. But definitely handling.

149. Being a dad means
upping your values a notch.
Maybe two or three notches.

•

150. Being a dad means getting
mother and child home and
realizing you're on your own.

•

151. Being a dad means taking the
week off after your baby comes home.

•

152. Being a dad means letting
your wife teach you child care.
One, it comes naturally to her, and,
two, she's read all the books.
You've read *Sports Illustrated.*

153. Being a dad means realizing that all the stupid stuff your wife bought to simply change the baby—like wet wipes, diaper pins, a lined trash can with a lid, new outfits, and diaper rash cream—are, well, really important.

•

154. Being a dad means teaching your baby two words: Da Da.

•

155. Being a dad means putting your child's wants, needs, and desires ahead of your own wants, needs, and desires. Every day.

156. Being a dad means looking at your baby all night the first night home.

•

157. Being a dad means making eye contact with your baby often.

•

158. Being a dad means strengthening your baby by gently moving her arms and legs up and down and in circles—and doing this every night. Babies and dads love this.

•

159. Being a dad means rocking your baby to sleep late at night. And talking to her the whole time.

160. Being a dad means deciding there's more sleep, more rest, and more sex if the baby sleeps in his own bed.

•

161. Being a dad means getting the baby out of your room as soon as possible. Even though you stay up all night the first night listening to the baby monitor.

•

162. Being a dad means not wanting to say, "Sippy cup" in public.

163. Being a dad means starting
a 529 college savings plan now.
Three hundred dollars a month will
turn into more than $110,000 in seven-
teen years. (That won't be enough.)

•

164. Being a dad means telling
grandparents that contributions
to the college fund will always
make nice birthday gifts.

•

165. Being a dad means holding
a peeing baby over the sink.

166. Being a dad means swearing
you'll never carry a diaper bag,
so you force all of its contents
into a duffel bag or briefcase.

·

167. Being a dad means realizing
too late what your briefcase
will smell like for two years.

·

168. Being a dad means coming
home exhausted, collapsing
into your easy chair, and then
wondering why your butt feels wet.

169. Being a dad means holding your baby upside down above your face. And getting drooled on.

•

170. Being a dad means finding yourself curiously reluctant to handle baby poop.

•

171. Being a dad means thinking the entire house smells of dirty diapers, so you make a substantial investment in room spray, carpet spray, even spray deodorant. Your wife, however, thinks you've lost your mind because she doesn't smell a thing.

172. Being a dad means taking nothing your wife says during postpartum personally. Hormonally, she's a whack job.

•

173. Being a dad means staging a baby formula taste test. Because you want to know.

•

174. Being a dad means asking women for help in a baby-changing room and then letting them change the diaper for you. And then taking credit for it.

175. Being a dad means tasting baby food because you know you've put worse things in your mouth and then deciding, no, you actually haven't. The kid's on her own.

•

176. Being a dad means dropping your baby off at the grandparents' house and taking your wife away for two or three days. You need it, she needs it, you both need it.

•

177. Being a dad means using Scotch tape on the diaper when the diaper strips don't do the job.

178. Being a dad means rocking your baby back to sleep at 2:00 a.m. while listening to your iPod.

•

179. Being a dad means feeling satisfied if the diaper doesn't fall off.

•

180. Being a dad means thinking a colorful baby mobile is eighty more dollars down the drain—until you realize it can buy you twenty extra minutes of sleep in the morning.

181. Being a dad means learning "colic" is shorthand for "screaming, unhappy baby, 3:00 a.m. rocking, worried sick, and exhausted parents."

182. Being a dad means realizing small children create a magical time in life. And praying you won't miss it.

183. Being a dad means thinking every now and then that you've bought everything a baby could possibly need for the next two years and that the money hemorrhaging will stop. Mothers, for some reason, never think this.

184. Being a dad means losing hair to little hands pulling on chest hair, nose hair, head hair, beard hair, and—the most painful—leg hair.

•

185. Being a dad means sharing with Mom the fact you think she's spending too much on baby food and diapers and clothes. And about sixty seconds later regretting you brought the whole thing up.

•

186. Being a dad means learning that talking about the baby will often put a new mother in the mood for sex. So you find yourself talking bottle warmers and booties at the oddest times.

187. Being a dad means
gently roughhousing with your
child even though the mother
thinks he will break. Babies love it.

•

188. Being a dad means deciding the
baby can only ride in the Mom Car so
that your car will not be abused with
puke, spilled baby formula, leaky
diapers, smelly car seats, and half-eaten
animal crackers stuck to the floor.

•

189. Being a dad means
resolving to spend time with your
child—real, meaningful, "I could
be on the golf course" and "I got
home from the office early" time.

190. Being a dad means semiconscious 3:00 a.m. feedings even though you used to be able to party all night.

191. Being a dad means wondering how such a tiny little baby can grin and deliver a nuclear blast in her diaper.

192. Being a dad means living with the feeling that you don't have the faintest idea what you're doing.

193. Being a dad means filling out the crush of medical and insurance forms that arrive from the hospital. It's daunting, but it'll save you money.

194. Being a dad means learning that babies cry when they're hungry. When they have gas. When they're tired. And, after a few weeks, when they're lonely.

•

195. Being a dad means accepting the fact that there are times you can't stop a baby from crying. And anger will only make things worse.

•

196. Being a dad means realizing moms can often stop a baby's crying faster than dads can. Don't take this personally.

197. Being a dad means thinking about hiring a nanny, even part-time, especially if you're traveling the first year.

•

198. Being a dad means surveying your once cool condo that's now besieged by Baby's bassinet, crib, diaper boxes, toys, stroller, car seat, and clothes. And deciding you like the new look.

•

199. Being a dad means telling the in-laws that a really good baby gift idea would be a high chair. (A good one can set you back $200.)

200. Being a dad means deciding baby talk is macho. Really. Dadagoogoo.

201. Being a dad means knowing that a crying or fussy baby could have made even Dr. Spock feel incompetent.

202. Being a dad means sleepwalking at the office because you're so tired from the nighttime feedings.

203. Being a dad means letting your wife decide about breastfeeding. It's her body, and NFL players have grown up on formula.

204. Being a dad means
thinking you have the hottest
Euro Stroller on the block.

·

205. Being a dad means challenging
another dad to a stroller race.
You do not share this with your wife.

·

206. Being a dad means wearing
a baby carrier. Yes, you look stupid,
but it can save you from rotator cuff
surgery years down the road.

·

207. Being a dad means giving
your wife nine months to recover from
the last nine months. She can get
exhausted just going to the mailbox.

208. Being a dad means being realistic about sex when your wife comes home from the hospital. How sexy would you feel if someone just pulled a human being from your gut?

•

209. Being a dad means putting away your golf clubs for a while. Your nights and weekends are now booked.

•

210. Being a dad means never, ever criticizing your wife's mothering abilities. Get up and lend a hand instead.

211. Being a dad means finding you suddenly have weird mood swings, uncharacteristic irritability, and feelings of hopelessness. Postpartum depression strikes guys too.

•

212. Being a dad means making a financial plan. A baby born today can cost over $750,000 when college is figured in.

•

213. Being a dad means singing your favorite music to your baby at night. And the great thing about babies is, they don't care if you sing the Beatles, Twisted Sister, or Garth Brooks.

214. Being a dad means marveling at how something so tiny can wake the dead.

•

215. Being a dad means having a staring contest with your baby.

•

216. Being a dad means pushing a jogging stroller six miles. And realizing that, one day, they'll outrun you.

•

217. Being a dad means falling asleep while your baby sleeps on your chest. This magic lasts a couple of years.

218. Being a dad means
resolving not to miss the smallest
details of your baby's life.

•

219. Being a dad means
convincing yourself that you
change just as many diapers as
your wife although studies indicate
you're not even in the ballpark.

•

220. Being a dad means
looking all over town for
just the right plush teddy bear.

221. Being a dad means learning
that the cost of good child care
can rival that of private schools.
And figuring out how to afford it.

•

222. Being a dad means learning if
a prospective child-care facility has
installed camera monitors that you can
watch online, then going to the office
and watching the video feed all day.

•

223. Being a dad means teaching
Sunday school or Temple school,
because that's where the best
baby-sitters come from.

224. Being a dad means feeling like your life means something when you get your baby to burp.

•

225. Being a dad means reassuring Mom the baby will still be alive if she leaves you alone with her for two hours.

•

226. Being a dad means learning how to comfort a screaming baby, not hand him off to Mom.

227. Being a dad means writing down everything that happens. You'll have incredible memories to visit ten years from now.

•

228. Being a dad means realizing a day with clients, meetings, business lunches, and conference calls sounds like a spa vacation to a mom at home alone all day with a fussy baby.

•

229. Being a dad means showing a six-month-old how to have fun with pureed carrots.

230. Being a dad means
learning strained beets don't
wash off white business shirts.

•

231. Being a dad means emerging from
the baby's bath wetter than the baby.

•

232. Being a dad means
reminding Mom the family can go
out to eat in the evening because
babies can sleep anywhere.

•

233. Being a dad means unloading
your briefcase at a meeting and
finding a pacifier. You never want to
be without one of those little suckers.

234. Being a dad means finding barf on your shoulder as you're walking into a client meeting.

•

235. Being a dad means your relationship with your wife is changing. Profoundly. It's no longer just about the two of you.

•

236. Being a dad means realizing when a baby comes, the in-laws do too.

•

237. Being a dad means seeing grandmothers as the best baby-sitting deal around.

238. Being a dad means
smiling and nodding when your
father-in-law says your baby looks
a lot like his side of the family.

•

239. Being a dad means
accepting the fact your home
looks like a day-care center.

•

240. Being a dad means
changing a baby on your lap while
you sit in a stall in the men's room.

•

241. Being a dad means
inexplicably dropping the
word *potty* into conversations.

242. Being a dad means putting
a baseball into your son's crib.

•

243. Being a dad means putting your
hand on your child's chest at night to
make sure she's still breathing.

•

244. Being a dad means thinking you'll
save money by buying diapers online,
but the plethora of brands, sizes,
shapes, materials, and deals sends you
to WalMart to buy whatever's on sale.

•

245. Being a dad means learning
to do things one-handed.

246. Being a dad means teaching your kids that food is a great thing to throw at one another. Before Mom gets home.

•

247. Being a dad means trying to read the paper with someone crawling up your leg. . . and using your leg hair as grips.

•

248. Being a dad means getting to know other men with babies. Your single friends have little support to offer here.

•

249. Being a dad means learning to trust your instincts. This will work well for the next thirty or forty years.

Toddler Dads

250. Being a dad means being your child's entertainment center.

•

251. Being a dad means watching the Muppets for free on YouTube.

•

252. Being a dad means knowing that God will help you be the father He wants you to be. Just ask.

•

253. Being a dad means wondering how you can run a company, yet fail to get a two-year-old into the bathtub.

254. Being a dad means learning the hard way that a two-year-old has more energy than you.

•

255. Being a dad means reading the newspaper to your kids at breakfast. One day they'll ask for the business section.

•

256. Being a dad means not hesitating to use the words *no, never, absolutely not,* and *because I'm your father.*

•

257. Being a dad means understanding that this could be the most hilarious time of your life.

258. Being a dad means being told Mom's cooking is better.

•

259. Being a dad means realizing that fatherhood is cool.

•

260. Being a dad means you may be the first adult your wife has talked to in ten hours.

•

261. Being a dad means giving piggyback rides on demand, but drawing the line at carrying three riders at once.

262. Being a dad means shocking yourself while showing a four-year-old what happens when you stick a screwdriver into a wall socket.

•

263. Being a dad means teaching your children that their body is their own and nobody can touch it without their permission. And if anybody does, they need to tell you.

•

264. Being a dad means buying a DVR. Ostensibly so you can record children's shows. In reality so you can watch your favorite TV show when your kids are asleep.

265. Being a dad means never trying to reason with anyone who poops in his pants.

•

266. Being a dad means letting your two-year-old start dismantling a department store display to see what happens first: the display gets demolished or a panicked salesclerk shows up to wait on you.

•

267. Being a dad means telling a child who refuses to eat not to eat.

•

268. Being a dad means working late and getting a tearful phone call saying she can't go to bed without a hug from you.

269. Being a dad means admiring scars rather than being alarmed by them.

•

270. Being a dad means teaching a boy to aim first, then pee.

•

271. Being a dad means explaining to your daughter she doesn't need to lift the seat to pee.

•

272. Being a dad means letting your child clean up the spilled milk. Think of this as a life lesson.

•

273. Being a dad means reading to your kids every night. Even if it's the sports section.

274. Being a dad means watching your kids have more fun with a box than with the $200 toy that came in it.

•

275. Being a dad means that reading time often develops into tickling time.

•

276. Being a dad means asking the teenage cashier with face jewelry if she baby-sits in her spare time.

•

277. Being a dad means trying to make a three-year-old understand that while it's okay to run around naked in the backyard, she needs to put something on before dashing out the front door.

278. Being a dad means taking whiny kids outside in the pouring rain to show them that rainy days are great fun.

•

279. Being a dad means watching your son eat a bug—and then eating one in front of him to make him howl.

•

280. Being a dad means showing your kids how to stomp on a spider. And telling them not to freak out over the crunching sound.

•

281. Being a dad means figuring out that if you have more than two kids, you're outnumbered. You have to shift from a man-to-man defense to zone.

282. Being a dad means losing HBO for about fifteen years because you don't want to have to worry about what your kids are watching.

•

283. Being a dad means making your child swim to you. Time and time again.

•

284. Being a dad means teaching your kids to face their fears. They'll watch how you face yours.

•

285. Being a dad means watching cartoons with your kids because you think one more visit to Mister Rogers' neighborhood could make you go postal.

286. Being a dad means testing your kids to be sure they know their first and last names, your name, their mom's name, and their address and telephone number.

287. Being a dad means teaching your kids when to call 9-1-1.

288. Being a dad means reading the dad blogs on the Internet and wondering if you would have liked those guys in high school.

289. Being a dad means thinking a new trike should contain six, maybe ten, pieces tops and it will be easy to assemble on Christmas Eve.

290. Being a dad means spending all Christmas Eve night putting together the five hundred pieces of new trike, while your wife keeps yelling from the bedroom that you should have paid the store to do it.

•

291. Being a dad means missing the football game to take your kids to a stultifyingly boring kids' movie—and having them fall asleep ten minutes into it.

•

292. Being a dad means wondering if day-care centers douse your kids in grape juice before sending them home.

•

293. Being a dad means playing catch with a ball covered in glitter.

294. Being a dad means taking
Cinderella or Spiderman
to McDonald's.

•

295. Being a dad means lying on the
couch with a handful of Advil after
doing somersaults with your children.

•

296. Being a dad means
regretting that you didn't teach
them that superglue is forever.

•

297. Being a dad means
spending Saturday mornings
in the doughnut shop reading the
paper while your kids inhale chocolate-
covered bear claws and Coke.

298. Being a dad means encouraging your kids to feel your muscles because your wife refuses to.

●

299. Being a dad means holding a smashed spider in your palm and telling a four-year-old to touch it.

●

300. Being a dad means convincing a hesitant child that it's fun getting launched off your shoulders into a swimming pool—and then hours later begging the same child to let you out of the pool because you are exhausted and need Advil.

●

301. Being a dad means telling your kids to get up when they fall.

302. Being a dad means looking at a skinned knee and saying, "Come back when you're really bleeding."

•

303. Being a dad means showing your son how to lick blood off his arm or leg when he scrapes himself.

•

304. Being a dad means showing your scars to your kids and telling them how much you bled in order to get them.

•

305. Being a dad means letting your child dress herself for preschool even if she emerges wearing a Batman costume.

306. Being a dad means lying in the grass with your child and finding shapes and faces in the clouds.

•

307. Being a dad means serving sweet rolls for breakfast every morning because kids will eat them. Besides, milk will balance everything out.

•

308. Being a dad means looking your three-year-old in the eye and telling her there's nothing scary about going to the dentist even though you haven't been in ten years because, well, thinking about it gives you nightmares.

309. Being a dad means
letting your kids drink Coke
at breakfast when Mom isn't
looking because it keeps them quiet
and they're going to school and the
teachers will be able to handle them.

•

310. Being a dad
means thinking Muppet
humor is really sophisticated.

•

311. Being a dad means trying
to get a three-year-old to
memorize the multiplication
tables by singing them to her.

312. Being a dad means having the unique ability to not hear a child's whining. Moms do not share nor appreciate this trait.

•

313. Being a dad means telling Mom you're not going to make the kids eat their Brussels sprouts because they make you gag too.

•

314. Being a dad means turning vacuuming into a game of chase.

•

315. Being a dad means building a fort. Out of a sheet.

316. Being a dad means realizing you spend more time at your desk than you do with your child.

•

317. Being a dad means making the tough decision that your toddlers are not old enough to use the remote control. Or even hold it. So you tell them it could burn their hand.

•

318. Being a dad means giving an exhausted four-year-old fisherman a ride on your shoulders back to the car while you also carry the fishing rods and gear.

319. Being a dad means saying,
"Go outside and practice."
Then lying down on the couch.

•

320. Being a dad means falling
asleep before the evening news
even though you had big plans
for fooling around with Mom.

•

321. Being a dad means telling
a four-year-old that we all must
set goals in life and that your
goal for her is medical school.

322. Being a dad means realizing a sick toddler is preparing you for raising a teenager: both are sullen, depressed, and needy.

•

323. Being a dad means being the answer man. And if you don't know the answer, you make it up.

•

324. Being a dad means reading books using funny voices that cause your kids to collapse in laughter.

•

325. Being a dad means taking your child into the toy store on his birthday and telling him he can keep everything he can grab in five minutes.

326. Being a dad means deciding for toddlers—who can't decide for themselves—if they want to go for a walk or if they're scared of the birds.

•

327. Being a dad means telling your kids that if they want to whine, go see their mom.

•

328. Being a dad means making sure cell phones, car keys, Blackberries, iPods, and wallets are not touched by hands covered with peanut butter and jelly.

329. Being a dad means
watching your child eat a worm
and pondering whether this is info
you want to share with his mother.

•

330. Being a dad means giving
your kids a spade and telling them
to go dig a hole every time you
go outside to work in the yard.

•

331. Being a dad means
smelling the Mom Car every
week to see if the leftover food, wet
clothes, muddy boots, pet hair, and
spilled milk have begun to ferment.

332. Being a dad means instituting the "No Throwing Up in Dad's Car" policy. And reviewing it regularly.

•

333. Being a dad means wanting to use Mom's car to rush a sick child to the doctor because of the "No Throwing Up in Dad's Car" rule, failing to secure usage, pleading with the child to adhere to the rule. . . only to watch it be shattered before reaching the end of your street.

•

334. Being a dad means setting the goal of being home for breakfast and dinner.

335. Being a dad means talking to your kids. All the time. The number of words your kids know has a direct impact upon their IQ.

•

336. Being a dad means sniffing your child, then sniffing your dog, and then deciding they've both been rolling in the same thing.

•

337. Being a dad means not tolerating one sliver, one ounce, one grain of disrespect. Take care of it now and the high school years will be significantly easier.

338. Being a dad means knowing that, after your hard day at work, at least one person in the world will be delighted to see you.

•

339. Being a dad means saying to quarreling siblings, "You guys work it out."

•

340. Being a dad means bonding over cookies and milk.

•

341. Being a dad means taking the training wheels off. In fact, that pretty much defines fatherhood.

342. Being a dad means putting a Band-Aid on a skinned knee while the mother cries that taking the training wheels off was your idea.

•

343. Being a dad means eating a pie made of Silly Putty.

•

344. Being a dad means turning the telephone sales call from India over to your four-year-old. Salespeople will quit calling.

•

345. Being a dad means turning off the lights, giving your kids a flashlight, and telling them a ghost story that makes them run to Mama.

346. Being a dad means
having a toddler walk past one
bathroom, into your bedroom,
around the bed, and throw up on you.

•

347. Being a dad means
insisting your kids wear a bike
helmet while you refuse to.

•

348. Being a dad means getting
kids excited by wrestling with
them—and then telling them to
calm down so you can rest.

349. Being a dad means spelling words to your wife when the kids are around. Then realizing the kids might be more literate than you thought.

•

350. Being a dad means having your child point out the sunset that you somehow missed.

•

351. Being a dad means taking your kids to the library. It teaches them it's a place for smart people.

•

352. Being a dad means wondering if you're saying no too much.

353. Being a dad means actually believing (at least temporarily) that if you buy this one more stupid thing, your child will quit belly-aching about wanting stuff.

•

354. Being a dad means calling your kids as you're on the way to the office if you had to leave before breakfast. It will make their morning.

•

355. Being a dad means standing in a conga line at the mall for two hours so your child can have a picture taken with Santa even though your Christmas spirit disappeared an hour earlier.

356. Being a dad means taping your kindergartener's concert instead of watching it. Then somehow erasing the tape before you get it home.

•

357. Being a dad means reading Dr. Seuss books to her every night instead of the business journals you really need to read.

•

358. Being a dad means putting your kids' songs on your iPod and letting them listen to it. Of course, if your toddler toddles out of the room with your iPod, you may never see it again.

359. Being a dad means forgetting their songs are on your iPod and having to work out to Raffi during lunch.

•

360. Being a dad means showing them how to feed a cow without losing any fingers.

•

361. Being a dad means taking your kids on a bug hunt.

•

362. Being a dad means giving them the Gun Talk. Whether you keep guns in your house or not, your kids need to know what to do around one.

363. Being a dad means teaching your kids how to hold and throw a rock so it will skip at least five times across a lake.

364. Being a dad means telling Mom she's too easy on the kids.

365. Being a dad means showing your kids why they shouldn't throw tennis balls up at the ceiling fan when the fan is on, and you wind up showing them all afternoon— or until Mom comes home.

366. Being a dad means taking your kids horseback riding. Even if the horse is a twelve-year-old mare, they'll remember riding a wild stallion.

367. Being a dad means saying not wearing a coat will toughen them up.

•

368. Being a dad means saying, "Go ask your mom."

•

369. Being a dad means teaching your values and morals now. Because by their teenage years, they are practicing whatever they've learned from whomever they learned it.

•

370. Being a dad means showing your kids how to find their way home.

School-Age Dads

371. Being a dad means dressing up as Great Chief Running Bear for your Indian Princess.

•

372. Being a dad means taking your kids hiking. Even if it's just through the woods across the street.

•

373. Being a dad means realizing your kids have created an avatar of you and you like it.

•

374. Being a dad means teaching your child to hold out her right hand and introduce herself. Careers have been derailed over this.

375. Being a dad means making your kids laugh like nobody else can.

•

376. Being a dad means not wanting to explain the lyrics of the song they heard.

•

377. Being a dad means sleeping outside with your kids in a tent. Then at 11:00 p.m. everyone giving up and going back inside.

•

378. Being a dad means teaching them how to do chin-ups. Then realizing that, well, you could use a little work.

379. Being a dad means encouraging individual creativity. Not squelching it because you don't understand it.

•

380. Being a dad means giving up drinking until the kids leave home.

•

381. Being a dad means giving the Homework Talk. No TV, no video games, no phone calls, no laughter, no jokes, no Cokes, only life-sustaining liquids until homework is done.

•

382. Being a dad means watching for your child's hidden gifts and talents to surface. And, as soon as you spot one, you hire a private tutor.

383. Being a dad means
challenging them to hit you
in the stomach. Until one day . . .

•

**384. Being a dad means buying
a new house because you want
to live in a better school district.**

•

385. Being a dad means taking
the family to the go-cart track
because you really want to drive one.

•

**386. Being a dad means making
sure everybody in the family
knows how babies are made.
And how not to make them.**

387. Being a dad means buying your kids a chemistry set and the first experiment you teach them is how to make blue fire.

•

388. Being a dad means telling your kids it's definitely not okay to express their feelings whenever they feel like it.

•

389. Being a dad means taking along a book on birds whenever you take your kids to the park. That way, instead of saying, "I have no idea what kind of bird that is," you say, "Let's look it up."

390. Being a dad means realizing the high school years will be much more enjoyable if good manners are enforced now.

•

391. Being a dad means encouraging your child to work things out without you.

•

392. Being a dad means having the power to define your kids' future by what you tell them now. If you tell them they are smart, they will believe you. If you tell them they are stupid, they will believe that too.

393. Being a dad means teaching your kids where to cross a stream. And that, in life, there will be a great many streams to cross.

·

394. Being a dad means announcing that the dog is starving since no one has fed him in three days. Then pushing the remote control button.

·

395. Being a dad means teaching your son chess. Mercilessly beating him three times a week. And continuing to play him after he starts beating you.

396. Being a dad means realizing college is only ten years away and you haven't saved a dime. The calculator at SavingForCollege.com will help you determine how much you have to put away each month.

•

397. Being a dad means teaching them how to ride a bus, take a train, and hail a cab. These are life skills they need to know.

•

398. Being a dad means feeling guilty about missing dinner.

399. Being a dad means explaining to kids that there are creepy people out there. On the streets and on the Internet. And if they meet one, come tell you.

•

400. Being a dad means teaching your kids that God is behind the science.

•

401. Being a dad means limiting your kid's computer access to only child-safe sites and chat rooms.

•

402. Being a dad means having your kids work on the computer in the den where everybody can see the screen. Even you. . .from the couch.

403. Being a dad means teaching your kids they'll meet bullies in the lunchroom, in a chat room, on the playground, even in the executive suite. And bullies hate to be stood up to.

•

404. Being a dad means stressing the importance of family. Over and over again.

•

405. Being a dad means teaching kids it's foolish to argue about something they can find the answer to on the Internet.

•

406. Being a dad means showing your children how to cook your grandfather's favorite chili.

407. Being a dad means having your child ask you if you know where you're going.

•

408. Being a dad means sending them to camp to "toughen them up." Your wife will think it's time to put you on medication.

•

409. Being a dad means showing off your skateboarding skills and winding up with your leg in a cast.

•

410. Being a dad means sitting in a movie theater with two dolls on your left, a teddy bear on your right, and a sleeping seven-year-old on your lap.

411. Being a dad means laughing at yourself in front of your kids. They'll learn they can laugh at their mistakes too.

•

412. Being a dad means knowing there's a game of catch waiting for you at home. And looking forward to it.

•

413. Being a dad means informing kids there is no clean underwear fairy. And they can't wear yours or mom's.

•

414. Being a dad means teaching them not to interrupt. Especially you. Or their mother. Or their teachers. Or even their siblings.

415. Being a dad means teaching kids that our soldiers deserve our love, gratitude, and prayers.

•

416. Being a dad means lecturing about money and how it's earned and how a lot of things need to be done around the house that you might be willing to pay for.

•

417. Being a dad means hearing how every other kid gets an allowance. Or more allowance. And not caring.

•

418. Being a dad means letting your kids beat you in a race until the day you want to show them who's the dad.

419. Being a dad means being legitimately outrun by a ten-year-old. And not knowing whether to feel pride or start taking vitamins.

•

420. Being a dad means introducing the concept of responsibility—and living it in front of your kids.

•

421. Being a dad means taking your kids into the voting booth with you.

•

422. Being a dad means explaining democracy at the dinner table. And how, for instance, the family is a dictatorship.

423. Being a dad means teaching that one of the biggest barometers of future success is the ability to practice delayed gratification.

•

424. Being a dad means teaching your kids that if anyone online asks for their real name or address or their mother's name, then come tell you so you can pound that person into the dirt. And they can watch.

•

425. Being a dad means requiring your kids to use child-safe sites such as imbee.com, ClubPenguin.com, Neopets.com, and Whyville.net.

426. Being a dad means recognizing when a child has been in cyberspace too long and it's time for her to rejoin the family.

•

427. Being a dad means taking the kids for a long walk in the woods and then idly wondering if you just might be, well, lost.

•

428. Being a dad means explaining to your seven-year-old that you forgot what poison ivy looks like and now you both know and please pass the calamine lotion.

•

429. Being a dad means test-driving a Corvette with an ecstatic copilot.

430. Being a dad means building confidence in your kids. And noticing that doing so curiously builds yours.

•

431. Being a dad means helping your child push past his fears.

•

432. Being a dad means realizing your kids have your mannerisms.

•

433. Being a dad means monitoring computer games, but lusting after the newest PlayStation.

•

434. Being a dad means staying up late at night practicing your kids' computer games so you can destroy them the next day. (Moms do not understand this.)

435. Being a dad means regularly talking with your kids about who they are. What they like. What they want to be.

•

436. Being a dad means, upon finding your child on an unauthorized chat-room site, breathing slowly, then typing, "You're now talking to the father who's going to hunt you down, cut your spine out, and then put you in jail."

•

437. Being a dad means telling stories about how you had to mow yards when you were six to earn money for college.

•

438. Being a dad means teaching that actions speak louder than words.

439. Being a dad means teaching that trust isn't given; it's earned.

•

440. Being a dad means thinking you've spawned another Louie Armstrong when some teacher says your child has perfect trumpet lips.

•

441. Being a dad means enforcing the rule "Grades come first."

•

442. Being a dad means confessing that, while you never learned the piano, it's important they do. And telling them they'll thank you for it in fifteen years.

443. Being a dad means learning your kids don't really care anything about your baseball card collection.

•

444. Being a dad means knowing who their best friends are. And what they're really like.

•

445. Being a dad means encouraging your kids to take cards off the Angel Tree so they'll learn about giving to others.

•

446. Being a dad means talking to other dads about raising kids rather than about the business deals you closed that day.

447. Being a dad means giving the "you're going to have to raise your game for middle school" speech.

•

448. Being a dad means turning into the kind of dad who thinks clothes for young girls have run off the rails. And being amazed you're now that kind of dad.

•

449. Being a dad means riding roller coasters with your kids until one day you realize that only idiots or kids would put their life in jeopardy like that.

•

450. Being a dad means trying to explain to a child why the speedometer goes up to 160 but the legal speed limit is 70.

451. Being a dad means staying
up at night searching the Internet
for answers to questions your
child asked but you couldn't answer.
Questions like, "Why is the sky blue?"

452. Being a dad means
showing your son how to use
a lawnmower. And planning for the
day when he will do it all by himself.
Of course this day never comes.

453. Being a dad means
giving boxing lessons.

454. Being a dad means teaching
that the way to deal with a school
bully is a quick right cross to the
nose and then a kick to the groin.

455. Being a dad means
sitting in the principal's office
explaining your child's actions.

•

456. Being a dad means competing
in a "hold your breath under water"
contest and realizing your kids would
rather drown than let you win.

•

457. Being a dad means being the
show-and-tell project at school.

•

458. Being a dad means not believing
your child is sick enough to miss
school unless you see blood or vomit.

459. Being a dad means knowing the most dangerously toxic place on earth is a second-grade classroom.

•

460. Being a dad means deciding—after you had to drive to soccer, to dance, to gymnastics, to piano, to tutoring, to art class, and then to karate— that your kids are overscheduled.

•

461. Being a dad means taking charge of your kids' character development.

•

462. Being a dad means reviewing your drug, sex, and alcohol policies with your kids—often. It's easier for your kids to take a stand when they know what yours is.

463. Being a dad means teaching your child to have a conversation without turning away from you. Eye contact is good too.

•

464. Being a dad means sitting with your kids while they do their homework.

•

465. Being a dad means encouraging friendships with kids who look and sound different.

•

466. Being a dad means spending more time with your kids than with the TV.

•

467. Being a dad means letting your child teach you what she learned in class that day.

468. Being a dad means calling family meetings even if everyone hates them.

•

469. Being a dad means announcing to your twelve-year-old that the privilege of driving will not hinge on turning sixteen, but on behavior, grades, and savings they've acquired.

•

470. Being a dad means telling your twelve-year-old son there's nothing to look at when he's standing in your bedroom flexing his muscles and asking you to look at them.

471. Being a dad means subtly trying to interject the Sex Talk while you're helping him study his vocabulary words for English.

•

472. Being a dad means explaining that you don't have to be great at something to enjoy it. Golf is an example. Most people suck at it but love it anyway.

•

473. Being a dad means realizing that whatever you drink or smoke or consume, your kids will want to drink or smoke or consume.

•

474. Being a dad means seeing glimpses of the adult your child could become.

Dads and Teenagers

475. Being a dad means commanding your kids' respect. And reassuring them of your love. At the same time.

•

476. Being a dad means remembering four words: It's just a stage.

•

477. Being a dad means knowing that this is the time when kids need their dad the most.

•

478. Being a dad means reminding everyone just who makes the rules. And doing so regularly.

•

479. Being a dad means setting dating rules. Really, really firm dating rules.

480. Being a dad means realizing your kids would rather be seen with their friends than with you right now. But they still want their allowance.

•

481. Being a dad means stressing that education is the currency of the well off.

•

482. Being a dad means thinking your daughter's clothes are too revealing.

•

483. Being a dad means showing your kids that the avenues of success rarely run through Hollywood, rapping, or sports.

484. Being a dad means encouraging your teen to take the hardest courses imaginable in school.

•

485. Being a dad means being talked into allowing a MySpace page because all your kids' friends are on it and only dorks don't have one and you'll be able to look at it anytime and they'll keep it private and you're thinking the last thing you want to raise is a dork.

•

486. Being a dad means wondering what happened to that happy child who used to think you hung the moon.

487. Being a dad means teaching
your daughter that if she has
something really important
to say, say it. Don't text it.

·

488. Being a dad means not
confusing closeness with leniency.

·

489. Being a dad means determining
that the mood of the house won't be
set by a spoiled teenager but by Dad.
Let the kids worry about your moods.

·

490. Being a dad means posting
an ad for military school on
the refrigerator and only saying
it's an education option.

491. Being a dad means laying down the consequences of certain behaviors as well as certain accomplishments.

•

492. Being a dad means knowing your kids' friends. Talking to them. Driving them around. It's amazing what teenagers in the backseat talk about.

•

493. Being a dad means reminding your kids that homework is done with their mind alert, the lights on, and the TV off.

•

494. Being a dad means letting your wife and kids have their secrets.

495. Being a dad means
dealing with the reality that
your wife and your teenagers are
experiencing significant shifts in
hormones at about the same time.

•

496. Being a dad means having the
Sex Talk. Often. The "I won't pay
for a baby" lecture doesn't suffice.

•

497. Being a dad means letting
your teen's friends know how the
combination of teenagers and drugs
and alcohol and sex makes you lose
your mind. They'll get the message.

•

498. Being a dad means watching your
kids go to their mother for money.

499. Being a dad means e-mailing your kids from the office and asking how the homework's going.

•

500. Being a dad means being told by your kids they won't be seen with you until you change out of your Bermuda shorts and black socks and open-toe sandals.

•

501. Being a dad means laying down an ironclad curfew. Expect complaints.

•

502. Being a dad means showing by example how to talk to teachers, salesclerks, mail carriers, and waitresses. You're shaping the way your kids will treat people in the future.

503. Being a dad means not wanting your kids to judge others by the car they drive even though you know a Porsche would complete you.

•

504. Being a dad means looking at the Chemistry 1 textbook and saying, "You're on your own."

•

505. Being a dad means waking up your teen every morning even though your actions are never appreciated. Feel free to use the intercom.

•

506. Being a dad means having the dreaded STD Talk and finding that your kids are not as embarrassed as you are.

507. Being a dad means regretting the time you missed watching your kids grow up. And knowing you'll never get it back.

•

508. Being a dad means realizing you haven't bought new underwear in three years, but your kids look like they've stepped off the pages of *GQ* and *Vogue.*

•

509. Being a dad means sometimes wounding your child unintentionally.

•

510. Being a dad means taking a thirteen-year-old to the mall on the thin hope he'll say more than three words to you—and having him spend all his time on his cell phone.

511. Being a dad means reminding your teens that the heavens will fall if they come downstairs on Mother's Day without a gift.

•

512. Being a dad means helping your kids set priorities. Some kids think a nice tan should be their top priority.

•

513. Being a dad means believing the middle school years of driving them all around the county was God's way of preparing you to beg them to take driver's training as soon as they're old enough.

514. Being a dad means, after much prayer and mental preparation, teaching your kids to drive. In their mother's car.

•

515. Being a dad means telling your teens what the steering wheel is for, what the brakes are for, where the headlights are. They think they know. They don't know.

•

516. Being a dad means testing them on red light, green light, stop sign, school zone. They don't know.

•

517. Being a dad means seeing your retirement fund go up in smoke so you can pay the automobile insurance premiums for teenage drivers.

518. Being a dad means getting your teens checked for color blindness after they run their third stoplight.

·

519. Being a dad means making sure they know how to drive in five o'clock traffic—in the pouring rain—before they get their license.

·

520. Being a dad means riding with them as they learn to drive because their mother refuses to.

·

521. Being a dad means ignoring your teen's pleas for a new Beemer while you research pre-owned tanks. You want your offspring surrounded by steel.

522. Being a dad means
telling your teens they can use
the car—but they can't listen to
the radio, they can't talk on their cell
phone, they can't have more than one
friend in the car, and they can't leave
their zip code. But have fun.

•

523. Being a dad means
buying your new driver a
premium membership to AAA.

•

524. Being a dad means
insisting on a gasoline budget.
Or offering the alternative: a job.

525. Being a dad means showing your kids how to change a tire even though you haven't changed one since your dad showed you how. Then, after thirty frustrating and futile minutes, you tell them not to lose AAA's phone number.

•

526. Being a dad means getting your teen to agree to call you before stepping into a car with a drunk driver. Especially if he is that driver.

•

527. Being a dad means checking your car every morning for any new dings.

•

528. Being a dad means telling your teens that they pay for damages. And sticking to that policy.

529. Being a dad means preaching
that while trouble awaits if they drink,
hell awaits if they drink and drive.

•

530. Being a dad means explaining
to a teenager over and over again
that your money is not their money.

•

531. Being a dad means seeing
on the floor a note from one of
your kid's friends, thinking about
respecting her privacy, then reading it.

•

532. Being a dad means acting
upon the information in that note.

533. Being a dad means listening to a teenager say, "You don't respect my privacy." Agreeing that, no, you don't. And explaining she's still in trouble.

•

534. Being a dad means having your kids believe you're incredibly lucky to have made it this far in life without their advice.

•

535. Being a dad means teaching your kids how to read the financial section of the newspaper.

•

536. Being a dad means buying each of your kids a share of stock to track in the financial section.

537. Being a dad means
using words like *GNP, profit,
earnings,* and *yield* at the dinner table.

•

538. Being a dad means setting an
example on how to handle money.

•

539. Being a dad means
explaining that whining won't help
anyone get money, but work will.

•

540. Being a dad means teaching
that everything goes on sale.

•

541. Being a dad means showing
your teen how to return stuff to the
store and get his money back.

542. Being a dad means having
final wardrobe approval.

•

543. Being a dad means reminding
a teenager to be grateful.

•

544. Being a dad means
thinking a high school prom
couldn't be that expensive. Then
learning the limo alone is $1,200.

•

545. Being a dad means
telling your teen she's done a good
job. When she's done a good job.

•

546. Being a dad means taking your
kids with you when you do community
service. They'll say how bored they
are. But they'll get the message.

547. Being a dad means teaching that selflessness is a cure for selfishness.

•

548. Being a dad means saying "thank you" to your kids. And "I'm sorry."

•

549. Being a dad means talking about how dumb your brothers and sisters are. And then realizing you're teaching your kids it's okay to think brothers and sisters are dumb.

•

550. Being a dad means letting your kids see you fight through disappointment and failure.

551. Being a dad means teaching your kids there's a season for everything.

•

552. Being a dad means having the Alcohol and Drugs Talk. Again. And often.

•

553. Being a dad means teaching your kids there's dignity in struggle.

•

554. Being a dad means teaching that overnight successes usually take about twenty years.

555. Being a dad means telling your kids not to speed, then getting a speeding ticket.

•

556. Being a dad means taking comedy defensive driving with your teenager because both of you got speeding tickets. And thinking, all in all, it was a pretty good time.

•

557. Being a dad means constantly reminding your kids that everything about Hollywood is fake. Especially the people.

558. Being a dad means catching yourself before you yell at another driver. The last thing you want to teach your kids is road rage.

•

559. Being a dad means discovering that your kids know more about street drugs than you do.

•

560. Being a dad means encouraging big dreams.

•

561. Being a dad means giving your teen *Rich Dad, Poor Dad*.

562. Being a dad means
staying up until they come home.
This is self-induced insomnia
doctors will never be able to cure.

•

563. Being a dad means
continually teaching the biblical secret
to financial security is giving away
10 percent of your wealth. Even if
that 10 percent is only five dollars.

•

564. Being a dad means
taking walks one-on-one. Walk
long enough and they'll start
telling you what's on their mind.

565. Being a dad means reminding your kids that the rich and beautiful people in magazines aren't as happy as they seem. Nor necessarily as rich and beautiful either.

•

566. Being a dad means stressing the importance of a college education. Not an Ivy League education.

•

567. Being a dad means understanding that your kids will treat you like you treat them.

568. Being a dad means continually talking with your kids about their future. Make them think about it. Tell them it's okay if their plan changes.

•

569. Being a dad means going into their rooms and looking at their memories of the childhood you gave them.

•

570. Being a dad means buying *The Official SAT Study Guide* and thinking this is the ticket to Harvard. Then you learn the cost of a Harvard education.

•

571. Being a dad means wondering what they are learning at school.

Dads and Vacations

572. Being a dad means buying a car specifically for car trips. And telling everyone they can't drink in it, eat in it, or do anything in it but watch the scenery.

•

573. Being a dad means announcing to the family, "We're going to take our time, enjoy the sights, maybe have a picnic on the way"—and then refusing to stop for sixteen hours because you want to get there.

•

574. Being a dad means saying, "Don't look at your brother for one hundred miles."

575. Being a dad means loading up the family in the car, telling the youngest to point in any direction, then heading that way for some hundred and fifty miles. See what's out there.

576. Being a dad means telling the family to not worry about money, then worrying about money the whole trip.

577. Being a dad means sitting agitated at a rest stop while the kids pee for the forty-third time since leaving home.

578. Being a dad means having your kids take all the pictures because you can't figure out the camera.

579. Being a dad means pointing out the scenery even though no one wants to be interrupted from their Game Boy, text messaging, and iPod.

•

580. Being a dad means spending $6,000 on a ski vacation, $10,000 on a trip to Europe, $5,000 on a trip to Disney World—and having your kids remember most fondly a trip to a state park that cost $212 including tips.

•

581. Being a dad means being blamed when flights are cancelled, roads are impassable, the weather is getting worse, and you haven't figured out a solution.

582. Being a dad means arranging bulkhead seats on airplane trips because you know the crush of kid stuff you will be bringing onto the plane.

•

583. Being a dad means buying an expensive video camera, seeing no reason to read the directions (because, hey, you're a guy), and somehow erasing all the video. But, thankfully, the sound is still there. So it's weird radio.

•

584. Being a dad means thinking $80-a-day kids' ski camp is a good deal as long as the instructors wear them out.

585. Being a dad means agreeing to be buried in sand from the neck down at the beach. And then watching your kids get distracted and wander off.

•

586. Being a dad means making sure the kids get their own room.

•

587. Being a dad means agreeing that your kids can bring their best friend on the next trip.

•

588. Being a dad means agreeing to go to Disney World. And once there, thinking you've entered the seventh circle of hell.

589. Being a dad means having everyone in the family run their hands over the Vietnam Memorial.

•

590. Being a dad means taking your kids to Pearl Harbor to stand above the USS *Arizona* so they'll see just how much freedom costs.

•

591. Being a dad means taking your family to Ground Zero, where the World Trade Center used to stand. And not saying anything.

592. Being a dad means driving twelve hours to what was advertised as a "luxurious mountain cabin" only to discover it's an outhouse with a small kitchen attached.

•

593. Being a dad means taking your kids fishing in a mountain stream where you insist the fish are biting and, after fours hours of serious complaints about catching nothing, trying to shift the conversation to the joy of being outdoors.

•

594. Being a dad means taking the kids hiking in the woods—and then having your wife scream at you because everyone could have been eaten by bears.

595. Being a dad means taking the whole family to New York City. Walking the local neighborhoods, taking the subway, seeing the Statue of Liberty, grabbing a Yankee game.

•

596. Being a dad means shelling out big bucks for a deep-sea fishing trip, but not four dollars for the over-the-counter seasickness medication because you think it's too expensive.

•

597. Being a dad means going to a fish farm where you're given bait, rods, and a stocked pond. You come home with happy kids and even some fish.

598. Being a dad means pulling your kids out of school to go on vacation because this is the only time your vacation schedule and your wife's intersect.

•

599. Being a dad means taking the kids parasailing—and Mom not talking to you for the rest of the day.

•

600. Being a dad means forgetting about all the screaming and yelling and fights in the backseat and thinking this trip was the best ever.

College Dads

601. Being a dad means
paying for college.

•

602. Being a dad means accepting
that even though you've spent
thousands and thousands of dollars
on softball leagues, soccer teams,
volleyball coaches, piano tutors, and
violin lessons, your kids are not going
to get any kind of scholarship.

•

603. Being a dad means
telling your kids college isn't for
everybody. But growing up is.

•

604. Being a dad means telling them
all the wild things you did in high
school. Now that they've graduated.

605. Being a dad means telling
your kids to read the college catalog.

•

606. Being a dad means realizing
that, in spite of nursery school,
kindergarten, six years of grade
school, two years of middle school,
and four years of high school,
they're totally incapable of filling out
a college form without Mom's help.

•

607. Being a dad means sitting at a table
with your 17-year-old watching Mom
write the college application essay.

•

608. Being a dad means insisting
you won't pay for beer or partying.

609. Being a dad means telling your kids they can go to any college they want until you realize some schools cost over $40,000 a year and some cost less than $10,000 a year.

•

610. Being a dad means stating that he who pays for college gets to choose.

•

611. Being a dad means being quite clear about sex for the next four years: Bring home a degree. Not a baby.

•

612. Being a dad means getting excited about the fact that hundreds of thousands of dollars in scholarships go unclaimed every year.

613. Being a dad means deciding it's easier to come up with $25,000 a year than it is to qualify for one of those unclaimed scholarships.

•

614. Being a dad means learning it costs $50 to apply to one college. And your daughter wants to apply to ten.

•

615. Being a dad means refusing to fund a four-year music appreciation degree.

•

616. Being a dad means reminding your kids that, in all reality, it doesn't matter what college they go to. They just need a degree.

617. Being a dad means nixing schools stocked with trust-fund kids. Misery awaits if you can't keep up.

•

618. Being a dad means putting off funding your 401K for four years. Maybe longer.

•

619. Being a dad means telling your daughter to pick a college not because her boyfriend is going there, but because it offers a degree she wants to major in.

•

620. Being a dad means Googling your kid's roommate if you don't know him.

621. Being a dad means
suddenly realizing on moving day
just how empty your house is.

·

622. Being a dad means
telling your kid that if it doesn't fit
in the car, it won't fit in the dorm.

·

623. Being a dad means telling your
son he can't pack too much underwear
and too many socks. Especially if he
washes clothes only once a month.

·

624. Being a dad means paying some
$3,500 for a campus meal ticket only to
have them say they're going to need meal
money because they'll be sick of the
student cafeteria by the fourth day.

625. Being a dad means telling your college student to guard that meal ticket as if it were a fake ID.

•

626. Being a dad means going to all the parent orientation meetings on campus and wondering if your son is at the freshmen orientations or working on his tan.

•

627. Being a dad means making sure your freshman can find her way around campus. And knowing that, after you leave, she still won't know where she is.

•

628. Being a dad means not realizing your daughter is moving into a coed dorm until she tells you the person next door is "hot."

629. Being a dad means bringing your tool kit when you visit in case you need to repair the dorm room.

630. Being a dad means giving the Dad Talk about how your kids are going to college to learn, not just to party. And knowing they tuned you out at the word *learn*.

631. Being a dad means encouraging your son to go to the campus Career Center the first week of his freshman year and to stay in touch with those people.

632. Being a dad means accepting their relationships with the opposite sex will now get a lot more complicated.

633. Being a dad means going to the campus bookstore and buying yourself a college T-shirt. Your kids beg you not to wear it around campus, but you do.

•

634. Being a dad means driving home in tears.

•

635. Being a dad means feeling like your family has been ripped apart. Even though she's only a couple hours away.

•

636. Being a dad means talking to other new college dads in hopes of feeling better, but they're as miserable as you are.

637. Being a dad means buying season tickets to the college football games. And learning later they didn't make it to a single game while you drove four hours every Saturday in order not to miss one.

•

638. Being a dad means putting your kids on a budget. And answering their requests for a new DVD, a new TV, a new computer, a new iPod, and new clothes with "That's why God created student jobs."

•

639. Being a dad means getting told that other parents give their kids more money.

640. Being a dad means telling them that selling their books for party money means they'll be living at home next semester and working full-time.

•

641. Being a dad means working twelve hours a day, driving a ten-year-old car, and taking out a second mortgage just to pay for college—and having your daughter tell you that school is killing her and she needs a vacation in Cabo.

•

642. Being a dad means understanding that no one is happy all the time. And kids between eighteen and twenty-two years have wild mood swings.

643. Being a dad means
trying to rationalize with
someone who uses a fake ID.

•

644. Being a dad means insisting
your kids take out a student loan to
pay for part of school. Especially if
studying harder in high school would
have reduced the cost of college.

•

645. Being a dad means
telling them you'll share your
college stories the day they graduate.

•

646. Being a dad means showing
up for Parents' Weekend only to
learn your kids have left town.

647. Being a dad means praying your kids won't act like you did in college.

•

648. Being a dad means reassuring them there's honor and glory in struggling for good grades on little money and sleep.

•

649. Being a dad means wondering if beer has become a major food group.

•

650. Being a dad means suggesting your kids start studying before 10:00 p.m. It's a useless conversation, but you'll feel better afterward.

651. Being a dad means knowing the reason a lot of college kids don't try cocaine is because they can't afford it. Which is one more reason you don't give them all the money they want.

•

652. Being a dad means encouraging your kids to get to know their professors and to talk to them regularly. Tell them not to wait until finals to do this.

•

653. Being a dad means giving advice when asked for money.

•

654. Being a dad means listening to your daughter talk all about her classes. Even when she's trying to explain why organic chemistry is cool.

655. Being a dad means realizing that if she calls in tears saying she hates college because she has no friends, she's just broken up with her boyfriend.

•

656. Being a dad means wanting to explore the reason they suddenly want to take acting classes.

•

657. Being a dad means encouraging them to join all the clubs relevant to their major. This is where contacts for future jobs are made.

•

658. Being a dad means being told she can't stand living in a dorm, that the coolest kids live in apartments.

659. Being a dad means
having conflicting ideas over the
purpose of summer. Your kids
will think it is to tour Europe on
your nickel, and you will think
they need to earn their own nickels.

•

660. Being a dad means having
political arguments with college
sophomores who get their
news from Comedy Central.

•

661. Being a dad means telling
your kids that if they need to drop a
course because they're failing, they will
pay for it out of their own pocket.

662. Being a dad means reminding them that college students who do summer internships are the ones who get jobs after graduation.

•

663. Being a dad means learning to dread two words: spring break.

•

664. Being a dad means being told how to dress by a college student. You'll have to remind her that looking twenty-two isn't your primary goal in life.

665. Being a dad means tossing down your stool softener about the time your daughter finishes doing her hair to go out for the night.

•

666. Being a dad means realizing they expect a big gift at graduation and telling them they just got a $100,000 present.

•

667. Being a dad means enjoying every moment of your student's graduation. They won't understand your giddiness.

668. Being a dad means gently breaking it to your college grad that he's not entitled to the same lifestyle he knew when he was in high school. He's about to enter the world of starting salaries.

•

669. Being a dad means giving the Job Talk. This is the talk where you say, "I'm not paying for anything anymore. So you need a job."

•

670. Being a dad means teaching that getting a job is a job itself. They'll want to spend the morning on their tan, you'll want them to work all day at getting hired.

671. Being a dad means
encouraging your kids to chase
their dreams. On their dime.

672. Being a dad means stating
that graduate school is a very adult
idea. And adults pay their way.

673. Being a dad means
finding an invoice from a traffic
lawyer addressed to your graduate
and deciding that they're
learning how the world works.

674. Being a dad means
listening to your college grads
complain that their first paycheck
doesn't begin to pay for their lifestyle.
And treasuring that moment.

•

675. Being a dad means reminding
your kids to never let time or distance
get between them and their friends.

•

676. Being a dad means teaching
your kids to not go into the future
without God. It's a very scary place.

Dads and Spiritual Matters

677. Being a dad means being trusted by God with the biggest responsibility imaginable: raising His child. And remembering He's right by your side each step of the way.

•

678. Being a dad means being the spiritual leader in the family. And that means attending worship services, seeking spiritual training, and having regular prayer time.

•

679. Being a dad means teaching that if your kids don't believe in God, they'll be all alone in the universe.

•

680. Being a dad means using your moral authority when it comes to TV, computer games, movies, and clothes.

681. Being a dad means having to explain death. Of a pet. Of a grand-parent. Of someone even closer.

•

682. Being a dad means sometimes going to bed scared. And realizing there's only one place to turn to.

•

683. Being a dad means deciding on what you believe spiritually. Because this will impact how you raise your family.

•

684. Being a dad means raising kids with love, patience, courage, and a firm belief that God is ultimately in charge.

685. Being a dad means teaching your kids that being good doesn't come naturally to people. That's when it's time to ask God to help.

•

686. Being a dad means striving to be a man of character.

•

687. Being a dad means teaching that hatred and brutality are within all of us. But both can be overcome.

•

688. Being a dad means teaching this truth: if we depend on our own strength and successes to feel good about ourselves, we'll be unprepared for the difficult days all of us inevitably face.

689. Being a dad means telling your kids all about their real Father.

•

690. Being a dad means talking about war. Why it's horrible. Why it's been around since Old Testament times. Why it still happens.

•

691. Being a dad means taking your kids with you to feed the hungry.

•

692. Being a dad means going with your kids on a mission trip to a third-world country.

•

693. Being a dad means teaching kids that when they feel the worst about themselves, they need to go out and serve other people.

694. Being a dad means insisting the family go to worship services. As a family.

695. Being a dad means noticing when your kids show kindness to others. And quietly commenting on it.

696. Being a dad means teaching your kids to laugh at their mistakes. Not dwell on them.

697. Being a dad means understanding every person has to make up their own mind about God. Even your kids.

698. Being a dad means knowing your child's greatest fear is that Mom and Dad will divorce. Resolve that this will never happen.

699. Being a dad means teaching your children that God is alive and working in the world today.

•

700. Being a dad means knowing your child's spiritual condition will determine the path he takes in life.

•

701. Being a dad means realizing you're never alone. No matter how alone you feel.

•

702. Being a dad means saying prayers at the bassinet. Then at the crib. Then at your child's bed.

703. Being a dad means teaching your kids the importance of living their faith when no one is watching.

704. Being a dad means getting slightly embarrassed by the number of gifts your kids open on birthdays and Christmas.

705. Being a dad means having your church, synagogue, or temple bless your baby. Make it a very special occasion.

706. Being a dad means teaching your child the Ten Commandments.

707. Being a dad means
teaching your children the books
of the Bible. Many 12-year-olds
have no idea where to find Genesis.

•

708. Being a dad means explaining
there's more to this world than this
world. And living in light of that truth.

•

709. Being a dad means
knowing a child has to experience
pain to grow. And letting him.

•

710. Being a dad means
telling a child she can figure out
a problem herself. Even though
you want to jump in and solve it.

711. Being a dad means teaching that a simple act of kindness can change another person's day. And sometimes our own.

•

712. Being a dad means remembering the big picture: your children won't remember or care whether they were bottle-fed or breast-fed, whether Mom had an epidural or a drug-free birth, or whether they made their grand entrance at home or in the hospital. They will remember the love in the family and the values their parents taught them.

713. Being a dad means being
the spiritual rock of the family. This
requires a supernatural Resource.

•

714. Being a dad means having every
member of the family take time to list
all the things they're grateful for.

•

715. Being a dad means
teaching that true happiness
depends on our thoughts.

•

716. Being a dad means teaching
that success isn't a guarantee or
a right. But a consequence. And
sometimes an undeserved blessing.

717. Being a dad means
reminding your kids that
confidence comes by overcoming.

•

718. Being a dad means asking
God for the strength to keep your
hands off your older kids' problems.

•

719. Being a dad means teaching
your kids to pray for their enemies.
They don't have to love them.
They don't even have to like them.
They just have to pray for them.

•

720. Being a dad means
teaching them the best way to
deal with conflict is to face it.

721. Being a dad means resisting the temptation to overindulge your children. This is how you prepare them for adulthood.

•

722. Being a dad means influencing your kids' ability to form healthy, happy relationships by having a strong and healthy relationship with them.

•

723. Being a dad means understanding that the moments you spend volunteering for neighborhood committees, church fund-raising, or political campaigning, you're, in effect, volunteering your entire family to live without you during those times.

724. Being a dad means realizing you can't talk to your children about faith and God unless you yourself are living a moral and spiritual life.

•

725. Being a dad means trusting God enough with your resources that you tithe back to Him, even if you don't have very much.

•

726. Being a dad means knowing that faith starts in the home. Not in the church.

•

727. Being a dad means doing all that you can so that your kids will believe they're significant.

Dad Fears

728. Being a dad means being deathly afraid you won't be able to pull this whole dad thing off.

•

729. Being a dad means realizing you have to provide not only financial support, but emotional and spiritual support as well. And wondering how in the world other men do it.

•

730. Being a dad means acting strong even when you feel like the air is being sucked out of your stomach.

•

731. Being a dad means worrying that what little disposable income there is will be going to disposable diapers.

732. Being a dad means being worried about losing your job but telling your wife everything is all right at the office.

•

733. Being a dad means worrying you don't have your kids in enough activities—and then worrying they'll each need a Blackberry to keep up.

•

734. Being a dad means worrying your child won't make the team if you don't hire a private coach.

•

735. Being a dad means always calculating how much the family needs to make it through the next month.

736. Being a dad means
fearfully imagining what it would
be like to raise your baby alone.

•

737. Being a dad means trying to keep
the fear of something bad happening
to your child just beyond your state of
consciousness. That fear never really
goes away. But it can be managed.

•

738. Being a dad means
worrying about whether
you can afford Christmas.

•

739. Being a dad means doing
everything humanly possible to never
disappoint your children. And forgetting that disappointment is inevitable.

740. Being a dad means imagining the worst when your wife or child is hospitalized. And learning a whole new meaning of "trusting God."

•

741. Being a dad means anxiously wondering if your children will make it on their own.

•

742. Being a dad means thinking you'll never figure out how to feed, bathe, rock, and change a baby. And thinking your wife suspects the same thing.

•

743. Being a dad means wondering how much time at work is too much time, but also wondering what would happen if the work didn't get done.

744. Being a dad means worrying you're going to run out of money. And your kid is only five.

•

745. Being a dad means looking at your kids' Christmas wish list and realizing their toys would cost more than your mortgage payment.

•

746. Being a dad means not being able to go to sleep until you hear your teen get home and the front door close.

•

747. Being a dad means helping your kids get their first job because you're more worried about their unemployment than they are.

Dads and Moms

748. Being a dad means taking time off. Sometimes even from being a dad.

•

749. Being a dad means remembering kids come and go. Your relationship with your wife shouldn't.

•

750. Being a dad means worshiping the ground your kids' mother walks on.

•

751. Being a dad means resting on the couch, convinced you do at least 50 percent of the housework. (Sorry, it's only about a third.)

•

752. Being a dad means being affectionate with your wife in front of the kids. They'll say they hate it. Kiss her again.

753. Being a dad means letting the frustrations of work stay there.

•

754. Being a dad means getting away together, just the two of you. Even if it's only for the weekend.

•

755. Being a dad means being grateful for Saturday morning cartoons.

•

756. Being a dad means insisting on one date night a week. Even if the baby-sitter costs more than the date.

•

757. Being a dad means showing your kids how a man is to treat a woman.

758. Being a dad means refusing to fight with your wife in front of the kids.

759. Being a dad means being on the same page with your wife about how kids should be raised.

760. Being a dad means putting a lock on the bedroom door.

761. Being a dad means insisting the children treat their mother with respect.

762. Being a dad means marveling at her ability to manage the household and children.

763. Being a dad means remembering that children need clothes and shoes and food and toys and all kinds of stuff—and that stuff costs money. Don't whine.

•

764. Being a dad means thinking your wife has an easy job taking care of the kids all day. Until the day she's sick and you have to do it. Then you think an army of nannies is the solution.

•

765. Being a dad means not caring one whit about Father's Day, but knowing Mother's Day requires gifts, flowers, cards, and lunch.

766. Being a dad means learning the hard way to never tell your wife she's acting like her mother.

•

767. Being a dad means accepting that your new friends will be the husbands of the mothers she hangs out with at playgroups.

•

768. Being a dad means telling your wife what a great mom she is. Often.

•

769. Being a dad means never criticizing her in front of the kids.

770. Being a dad means being treated differently by your kids than the way they treat their mom. And understanding that's a good thing.

•

771. Being a dad means understanding you will have no help teaching your kids to face adversity. A mother's instinct is to protect them from adversity.

•

772. Being a dad means driving the kids around in the afternoon even though you've had a difficult day because your wife needs an afternoon off.

773. Being a dad means listening to her at night when she talks about who your kids will marry. Even though they're only in middle school.

•

774. Being a dad means understanding she's happiest when she's surrounded by her family.

•

775. Being a dad means agreeing to a family picnic because there's a genetic reason moms like them. Even though there are ants, mosquitoes, and no TV.

•

776. Being a dad means telling her not to spend so much money on the kids. Over and over and over and over and over again. It's useless.

Dads and Sports

777. Being a dad means agreeing
to coach a sport you know nothing
about because it's the only way your
child will get on a YMCA team.

778. Being a dad means cheering
over your kid's first home run.
But teaching that a successful life is
made up of hitting a bunch of singles.

779. Being a dad means putting
a hoop in the driveway with
the full knowledge that one day
your kid will beat you like a drum.

780. Being a dad means
destroying your kids at Wiffle
ball and explaining to your wife that
kids need to deal with competition.

781. Being a dad means reviewing the intricacies of the double steal with a six-year-old who just wants to play catch.

•

782. Being a dad means painting your stomach purple and standing shirtless in January while you yell for your child's team.

•

783. Being a dad means convincing yourself your child has tremendous college potential though she's only seven years old.

•

784. Being a dad means realizing what really matters to a team of five-year-olds are the cookies and drinks after the game. They don't care who won.

785. Being a dad means feeling guiltier over missing a game than a parent-teacher conference.

•

786. Being a dad means thinking your child will land on a shrink's couch because you missed a third-grade volleyball game.

•

787. Being a dad means suffering anxiety, night sweats, panic attacks, and short-term memory loss during your child's tryouts.

•

788. Being a dad means learning your pain is not your child's pain. If his failure to make the team bothers you more than it does him, it's time to reevaluate your priorities.

789. Being a dad means taking your dainty little princess to a hockey game and learning she loves all the hitting.

•

790. Being a dad means telling your kids which team to cheer for. They'll buy this when they're young.

•

791. Being a dad means taking your baseball glove to a major league game and telling your skeptical wife you want to catch one for the kids.

792. Being a dad means
being your child's first coach.

•

793. Being a dad means discovering
that playing with your kids as they
get older makes you play harder.

•

794. Being a dad means jogging
with your kids and realizing
they're showing you mercy.

•

795. Being a dad means telling
your kids to go to bed early because
they have a game tomorrow.

796. Being a dad means leaving
the office early to play catch.

•

797. Being a dad means
giving pep talks.

•

798. Being a dad means paying for
ski lessons to keep a six-year-old out
of your hair—and learning at the
end of the week that he flew down
a double–black diamond while you
were inching down the bunny slope.

•

799. Being a dad means tumbling
down a mountain and losing skis,
poles, gloves, and glasses because you
stupidly agreed to race your kids.

800. Being a dad means grudgingly realizing you can't keep up with them. As the doctor sets your leg.

•

801. Being a dad means telling your daughter she can be more than a cheerleader.

•

802. Being a dad means letting your kids turn you into a sportsman.

•

803. Being a dad means standing on the sidelines and knowing it's as far as you can go. This pretty much explains fatherhood.

804. Being a dad means
buying a soccer ball and asking
your child to autograph it.

•

805. Being a dad is teaching your
kids not to argue with the referee or
they'll never get the close calls.

•

806. Being a dad means
cheering for your older child
on one side of town while your
wife cheers for the younger one
in the next county. All weekend.

807. Being a dad means justifying the cost for making a premier soccer, baseball, or volleyball team as a way to land a scholarship.

•

808. Being a dad means realizing, years later, the odds of an athletic scholarship were slim and none.

•

809. Being a dad means reminding them to never take their eye off the ball.

Dads and Work

810. Being a dad means
knowing what your child looks
like sleeping but not eating, playing,
or dancing. Because you work from
5:00 a.m. to 8:00 or 9:00 p.m.

811. Being a dad means constantly
weighing where your time can
most benefit your family.

812. Being a dad means saying your
family is the most important thing in
the world to you. Then wondering if
that's why you work fifteen hours a day.

813. Being a dad means seeing your
kids maybe twenty minutes a day
during the week. On good days.

**814. Being a dad means
realizing the only place you can
read the newspaper is at work.**

815. Being a dad means not tucking your
kids into bed for three weeks because
you've worked till 8:00 p.m. every night.

**816. Being a dad means excusing your-
self from an out-of-town business dinner
so you can call home to say good night.**

817. Being a dad means staring
at the picture of your kids on your
desk and realizing it's five years old.

**818. Being a dad means
regretting that you haven't
spoken a word to your child today.**

819. Being a dad means
coming to grips with the fact that
children can be career killers.

•

820. Being a dad means keeping
some news to yourself. Like the fact
your company is laying off people.

•

821. Being a dad means interrupting
a meeting to pick your child up at
the child-care center—and feeling
glad that Mom couldn't do it.

•

822. Being a dad means
wondering if your kids are
proud of what you do for a living.

823. Being a dad means realizing your kids have no idea what you do all day.

•

824. Being a dad means meeting your child in the school cafeteria for lunch. And bringing McDonald's.

•

825. Being a dad means knowing you've achieved something special when you have work and family in balance.

•

826. Being a dad means taking your kids to work with you to prove you don't read the *Wall Street Journal* all day. But of course they find it on your desk.

•

827. Being a dad means taking the afternoon off to take your daughter to a museum.

828. Being a dad means understanding that a promotion means even less time at home.

•

829. Being a dad means coming home from work, eating dinner with your kids, kissing them good night, then going back to work.

•

830. Being a dad means realizing that putting the family first means sometimes you have to put work first.

•

831. Being a dad means not wanting to ask HR about family- friendly policies for fear of jeopardizing future advancement.

832. Being a dad means explaining to a child with a fever, a cough, and a runny nose how much fun she'll have at day care exposing others. Because neither you nor Mom can miss work.

•

833. Being a dad means not letting your work define you. You're more than an accountant for an international corporation. You're a dad.

•

834. Being a dad means parking your work in some remote corner of your brain as you head home. When you're with your kids, be with your kids.

835. Being a dad means teaching your kids there's honor in hard work. Whatever it is. That a waitress deserves as much respect as a CEO.

•

836. Being a dad means discussing the ups and downs of your career with your kids as they get older. So they'll remember you overcame struggles to get where you are.

•

837. Being a dad means telling people what to do all day—and then having a three-year-old tell you what to do on the weekend. That's why you're sitting on the floor in a stupid Superman cape.

Dads and Money

838. Being a dad means teaching your teens to live below their means.

•

839. Being a dad means teaching that almost everything can be had for less. It just requires patience and negotiations.

•

840. Being a dad means having the Money Talk. This is the talk where you tell your kids they have to start earning money, and they try to talk you out of it.

•

841. Being a dad means realizing you'll never be able to give your family everything they want. A lot of things maybe. But not everything. And that's no reason to feel guilty.

842. Being a dad means being a financial role model. If your kids see you being responsible with money, they will be. If they see you MasterCarding jet skis and big screens, they will wind up in credit counseling.

•

843. Being a dad means teaching delayed gratification. That Beemers and condos come to those who work, save, and wait.

•

844. Being a dad means realizing you're going to have to pay somebody to mow the yard despite the fact that you have healthy teenagers living at home.

845. Being a dad means being told by kids who do as little as possible for an allowance that they are being underpaid.

•

846. Being a dad means pointing out that, with free room, free food, free use of the big screen, free handling of the remote, plus free spending money, they're living in the top 1 percent of the world.

•

847. Being a dad means comparing yourself to what the dads on TV make.

•

848. Being a dad means learning that Mom is slipping them money under the table—and being okay with it.

849. Being a dad means computing that entire families have lived on less than what your family's automobile insurance premiums cost.

850. Being a dad means facing the dilemma of saving for retirement right about the time college tuition bills start arriving.

851. Being a dad means worrying your kids have it too easy. But being grateful to God that they do.

852. Being a dad means teaching your kids to pay their bills on time.

853. Being a dad means announcing that most millionaires spend their money on land and stocks, not Beemers and Rolexes.

•

854. Being a dad means teaching a high schooler to handle credit cards as if they're radioactive.

•

855. Being a dad means teaching financial literacy. Use terms like *profit*, *loss*, and *buyout* at the dinner table.

•

856. Being a dad means teaching your kids that regularly putting money into a savings account is a surefire way of getting rich.

857. Being a dad means
buying your teen a subscription to
the *Wall Street Journal* and insisting
she discuss the articles with you.

•

858. Being a dad means pointing out that
you can't tell who is truly rich just by the
car they drive or the clothes they wear.

•

859. Being a dad means helping your
kids understand that buying $10 cock-
tails doesn't add up to early retirement.

•

860. Being a dad means teaching
them that if they live on 125 percent
of their salary, it doesn't matter
how much they make—they're poor.

861. Being a dad means showing your kids that a percentage of their money should be used to glorify God.

•

862. Being a dad means telling them to do what they love. Satisfaction will follow.

•

863. Being a dad means teaching the biblical truth that with God's blessings come much responsibility.

•

864. Being a dad means continually trying to convince your kids that you're not rich.

Dads and Problems

865. Being a dad means being there when your kids really need a dad.

●

866. Being a dad means knowing the teen years are . . . well . . . weird.

●

867. Being a dad means knowing that boys use drugs to get high, and girls use drugs to lose weight or gain confidence.

●

868. Being a dad means realizing there's a definite line between trusting your kids and being an idiot.

●

869. Being a dad means curiously feeling like other adults are blaming you if your teenager is having problems.

870. Being a dad means popping on the iPod to hear what your thirteen-year-old is listening to. And thinking, *HE'S LISTENING TO THAT?!?!?*

•

871. Being a dad means noticing when she can't seem to make it down to breakfast on time. And going upstairs to find out why.

•

872. Being a dad means dealing with your children's problems as they happen, not just hoping things will get better.

•

873. Being a dad means insisting that everyone in the family be treated with respect.

874. Being a dad means giving your kids a glimpse of the inferno when they use foul or abusive language with you or their mother.

●

875. Being a dad means teaching them from a very young age that the very worst thing they can lose is your trust.

●

876. Being a dad means spending all summer with teenagers in the house because you've grounded them.

●

877. Being a dad means knowing alcoholics and addicts—even ones who share your last name—will walk across the street to tell a lie.

878. Being a dad means enforcing house rules. Your house rules.

•

879. Being a dad means knowing your authority will be tested. Expect it.

•

880. Being a dad means finding marijuana cigarettes in your kid's room and wondering how your father might have handled it.

•

881. Being a dad means monitoring your child's computer usage from your office.

•

882. Being a dad means learning who your kids' role models are. Heroin-using models? Time for a talk.

883. Being a dad means drug-testing your teen if necessary.

•

884. Being a dad means making your kids think you're angrier than you really are.

•

885. Being a dad means reminding your daughter that a cell phone, acrylic nails, the tanning salon, makeup, the car, and credit cards are privileges. That can be lost.

•

886. Being a dad means telling your son how to talk to a judge—unless he's just dying to go to the Big House.

887. Being a dad means
sitting down with your kid's favorite
video game and doing a body count.
Perhaps it needs to disappear.

•

**888. Being a dad means
listening to all sides without
judging. Then learning the facts.**

•

889. Being a dad means
wondering if you're the problem.

•

**890. Being a dad means
praying for guidance. Daily.**

•

891. Being a dad means
realizing threats mean nothing.
Consequences mean everything.

892. Being a dad means giving your kids enough rope to rebel without letting them hang themselves.

•

893. Being a dad means realizing your child's been talking for twenty minutes and you have no idea what she's said.

•

894. Being a dad means paying attention to your child's body— to eyes, posture, skin, and breath.

•

895. Being a dad means teaching your values and morals to your kids when they're young. If you wait until they're teenagers, you've waited too long.

896. Being a dad means teaching kids to tell the truth by your example.

•

897. Being a dad means telling your teens they can't date anybody over twenty-one . . . until they're over twenty-one.

•

898. Being a dad means praying your kids learn their actions have consequences before they get older and the consequences are more severe.

•

899. Being a dad means calling any parent you've heard is providing teens with alcohol and telling them you're going to sue.

900. Being a dad means
laying down the law and then
dealing with teenagers who are
skilled at finding loopholes in it.

•

901. Being a dad means
refusing to buy your teen a radar
detector—and not letting him
buy one for himself. The idea is
to stay alive during the teen years.

•

902. Being a dad means not saying
everything you'd like to say in the heat
of the moment. But going out for a
short run. Or a five-mile run. Maybe
a ten-mile run if you're really mad.

903. Being a dad means being consistent. With your love. With your discipline. Kids look for reasons to become confused.

•

904. Being a dad means knowing the difference between standing by your child and approving of their actions.

•

905. Being a dad means listening to your kid's dreams, desires, hopes, worries, fears, problems, and conflicts. Without comment.

906. Being a dad means saying truthfully that a lot of kids who have problems in the teenage world do fine in the adult world. They just had a rougher start.

•

907. Being a dad means taking pride when your child does the right thing.

•

908. Being a dad means giving your child the chance to earn back your trust.

•

909. Being a dad means being a source of hope.

Divorced Dads

910. Being a divorced dad means knowing your divorce just destroyed your child's safe, secure world.

•

911. Being a divorced dad means learning how much you miss coming home to smiles and hugs.

•

912. Being a divorced dad means remembering you're not Mr. Mom. You're Dad.

•

913. Being a divorced dad means realizing your fathering job isn't done. It's just gotten harder.

914. Being a divorced dad means establishing rules of behavior in your house. Which may be different from the rules in their mother's house. And that's the way it is.

•

915. Being a divorced dad means vowing to stay on top of paying child support.

•

916. Being a divorced dad means living close to your kids so they'll know you're not abandoning them.

•

917. Being a divorced dad means trying to keep as much as possible about your kids' lives the same because they suddenly have a fear of change.

918. Being a divorced dad means understanding that no matter what happened between you and your wife, the kids will blame themselves.

•

919. Being a divorced dad means calling your kids every night.

•

920. Being a divorced dad means not asking questions about their mother.

•

921. Being a divorced dad means turning your child's future over to the Father.

922. Being a divorced dad means
refusing to speak ill of your
kids' mother, no matter what
a pain in the side she might be.

•

923. Being a divorced dad
means convincing them—
despite all the damning evidence—
just because they lost one parent,
it doesn't mean they'll lose two.

•

924. Being a divorced dad
means realizing your kids are now
watching how you date and handle
relationships with other women.

925. Being a divorced dad means not introducing every woman in your life to your kids. Wait until about the tenth date.

•

926. Being a divorced dad means not farming the kids out on "visitation" days. They don't need to watch your TV with a baby-sitter. They need to be with you.

•

927. Being a divorced dad means always assuring your kids that you love them. And that you will always be there for them.

928. Being a divorced dad means agreeing with your former wife that the kids keep the house and the parents take turns living there.

•

929. Being a divorced dad means getting a call from the school about your daughter's grades and wondering what you can do about it since she lives with her mother.

•

930. Being a divorced dad means dealing with your wife's new husband and your child's new father figure.

•

931. Being a divorced dad means missing your kids terribly.

932. Being a divorced dad means wanting to be there for the difficult times as well as the good times.

•

933. Being a divorced dad means keeping a vigilant eye out for signs of depression, eating disorders, or any significant change in appearance or attitude.

•

934. Being a divorced dad means assuring your kids that it isn't their fault, that you and their mother were the immature ones.

•

935. Being a divorced dad means continuing to discipline them when necessary.

936. Being a divorced dad means finding out that as they get older, your kids might want to live with their mother.

•

937. Being a divorced dad means treating any time you have alone with your kids as sacred.

•

938. Being a divorced dad means realizing your kids must lean on you, not you on them.

•

939. Being a divorced dad means telling your kids that they can't do anything at all to get you and their mom back together. That they just need to be kids.

940. Being a divorced dad means putting your testosterone on hold. No overnight guests.

•

941. Being a divorced dad means putting the kids' needs first in spite of having to make difficult compromises with their mother.

•

942. Being a divorced dad means being more than a Disney-land Dad who just shows the kids fun and games and leaves the hard parenting to Mom.

943. Being a divorced dad means going to all the plays, concerts, soccer games, and PTA events. They need you to be active in their lives even if you're just in their lives part-time.

•

944. Being a divorced dad means not making the kids choose sides.

•

945. Being a divorced dad means insisting your kids love their mom.

•

946. Being a divorced dad means putting your kids' happiness ahead of yours. Which means they're more important than any new relationship.

947. Being a divorced dad means realizing they will feel jealous of new women and new kids in your life.

•

948. Being a divorced dad means showing them love even when they're showing you anger, resentment, and rebellion.

•

949. Being a divorced dad means getting counseling if necessary.

•

950. Being a divorced dad means wishing everything could have been different.

Stay-at-Home Dads

951. Being a stay-at-home
dad means deciding it takes a man
to do what has been, for thousands
of years, a mother's job.

•

952. Being a stay-at-home dad
means knowing the new lingo
of SAHD, WAHD, and WIHF.
If you don't know what any of this
means, then you're not one of them.

•

953. Being a stay-at-home dad
means answering the question,
"Where's Mommy?" all day long.

954. Being a stay-at-home dad means talking to clients over the phone and aiming the remote control at *Shrek* while your toddler crawls into your lap.

•

955. Being a stay-at-home dad means kissing your wife good-bye and then doing the dishes.

•

956. Being a stay-at-home dad means knowing that days filled with marketing meetings, interoffice politics, and sales quotas are a cakewalk compared to days filled with diaper changes, shopping, holding on to a squirming six-month-old, and temper tantrums.

957. Being a stay-at-home dad means throwing dirty diapers on top of your ego.

•

958. Being a stay-at-home dad means not being able to share the good news about a Swiffer WetJet with just any man.

•

959. Being a stay-at-home dad means being asked what you do all day.

•

960. Being a stay-at-home dad means being asked by other women if you dressed your children.

•

961. Being a stay-at-home dad means realizing a good part of the locker room can't identify with you.

962. Being a stay-at-home dad means taking your child to a play-group and having soccer moms regard you as either a pervert or a hero.

•

963. Being a stay-at-home dad means having diaper companies send you a personal e-mail wishing you "Happy Mother's Day."

•

964. Being a stay-at-home dad means talking to your wife regularly about how she feels about being the breadwinner.

965. Being a stay-at-home dad means feeling unappreciated by your wife when she isn't home in time for dinner.

•

966. Being a stay-at-home dad means realizing you're an excellent father.

•

967. Being a stay-at-home dad means wondering how you could explain this gap on your resumé should your marriage end in divorce.

•

968. Being a stay-at-home dad means being able to truthfully say, "The most important things to me are my kids."

Parting Words

969. Being a dad means raising your kids to live without you.

•

970. Being a dad means learning the fine art of letting go.

•

971. Being a dad means telling your kids they can go to Los Angeles or New York to chase their dreams—but they pay.

•

972. Being a dad means asking your kids how their prayer life is.

•

973. Being a dad means being amazed at what your child has become. And telling him so.

974. Being a dad means threatening your kids with the reminder that one day they'll be taking care of you.

•

975. Being a dad means calling your business friends and asking them to interview your college graduate.

•

976. Being a dad means being a mentor.

•

977. Being a dad means fondly remembering the four-year-old your child once was. And admiring the adult she's become.

•

978. Being a dad means telling your adult kids you were already married and settled down when you were their age.

979. Being a dad means
helping them set realistic expectations
after graduation. Like the fact that
they don't need a Lexus. They need
an apartment and a car that runs.

•

980. Being a dad means urging your
kids to make the world a better place.

•

981. Being a dad means
telling your children there are
second chances. And giving them.

•

982. Being a dad means giving
your kids challenging books to read:
business books, financial books,
great literary classics.

983. Being a dad means teaching that seeing isn't believing. But believing is seeing.

•

984. Being a dad means reminding your kids to not be afraid of failure. That a lot of the world's most successful people experienced failure time and time again.

•

985. Being a dad means breaking the myth about glamorous jobs: they're hotly competitive, they pay the least, and they are the hardest to earn real money doing. Show them your electrician's house.

986. Being a dad means telling
your kids they will be responsible for
any new life they bring into the world.

•

987. Being a dad means
encouraging your kids to travel,
to see the countries whose names
they can barely pronounce.

•

988. Being a dad means
reminding them of their gifts.

•

989. Being a dad means teaching your
kids that they can be an instrument of
God by helping those less fortunate.

•

990. Being a dad means not
expecting any thank-yous.

991. Being a dad means
you will every now and then
pick your kids up, dust them off,
and send them back into the game.

•

992. Being a dad means quietly
thanking God when you learn they're
going to church on their own.

•

993. Being a dad means explaining
that the average life span is long
enough for people to succeed in a
number of different careers.

•

994. Being a dad means
teaching your kids that the most
valuable asset they can have as they
enter the adult world is their integrity.

995. Being a dad means encouraging your kids to live fearlessly.

•

996. Being a dad means having your college freshman call you, thinking you're about to have a nice conversation, and then suddenly hearing, "Gotta go!"

•

997. Being a dad means extending grace for the past.

•

998. Being a dad means reassuring them that 90 percent of the things they're most scared about will never happen. And God will give them the power to deal with the rest.

999. Being a dad means
encouraging your kids
to live for a noble cause.

•

1000. Being a dad means teaching
them that happiness is something
that happens while striving for
honor, living with integrity,
and serving God.

•

1001. Being a dad means
telling them they are the
kids you always wanted.